"In *6 Steps To A Healthier You*, Deborah Lobart inspires you to open your heart and look beyond healthy food and working out to achieve optimum health. She encourages you to go within to uncover what true happiness, peace and joy feels like by implementing simple foundational wellness practices that we so often neglect in our busy world.

You'll find yourself thinking, "that's me," countless times as she shares her story as a busy mom—running a business and raising children—whilst navigating her health issues and in the process re-aligning herself to a more grounded, purposeful and healthy way of life.

Her honesty and transparency will nourish your soul with light bulb moments hidden within each chapter that reveal insights that shift you to reflect upon your own life.

This book is easy to read and implement with questions at the end of each chapter taking your journey from information to transformation through reflection and action.

Deborah embodies what she teaches. Her extensive leadership, mindset, and business expertise as well as sound health guidance based off her journey of healing will provide you with wisdom that enriches your own life.

This book is a must-have for every mother who finds herself caught up in "busyness" and knows that something needs to change."

—**Debbie Spellman**, Mom, Coach & Speaker

6 STEPS TO A HEALTHIER YOU

A Mom's Healing Journey From The Inside Out

DEBORAH LOBART

BALBOA.PRESS

A DIVISION OF HAY HOUSE

Balboa Press books may be ordered through booksellers or by contacting:

Balboa Press
A Division of Hay House
1663 Liberty Drive
Bloomington, IN 47403
www.balboapress.com
1 (877) 407-4847

Print information available on the last page.

ISBN: 978-1-9822-5054-6 (sc)
ISBN: 978-1-9822-5056-0 (hc)
ISBN: 978-1-9822-5055-3 (e)

Library of Congress Control Number: 2020912038

Balboa Press rev. date: 07/25/2020

CONTENTS

This book is dedicated to the busy moms.
Wishing you health, happiness,
and fulfillment—

Deborah

THANK YOU

First and foremost, thank you to my husband Adir for constantly being there through thick and thin and always supporting me on my journey. If it weren't for you, none of the struggles that I have overcome would have been possible.

Thank you to my beautiful children Gabriella and Bobby for teaching me to live in the present. You have given me fulfillment beyond what I ever dreamed was possible. I promise to always support you in living your best life - I love you, unconditionally.

Thank you to my mom and dad for your endless love, support and always telling me to reach above and beyond; and, my siblings for the ongoing encouragement whenever I needed it most.

And of course, a big thank you to the countless coaches, healers and doctors who have been instrumental in my healing journey. I have learned so much from all of you and I am eternally grateful.

My goal is not to be better than anyone else, but to be better than I used to be.

Wayne Dyer

INTRODUCTION

When I was scrambling for ideas on how I was going to write this book, one thing remained certain. I wanted to create a book that I wish I had as a new mom - one that talks about *all* the elements of living a healthy lifestyle. Because as someone who was always health conscious—I thought I had it figured out. I believed that if I was just taking care of my physical body then I was doing enough. But as you'll soon find out, that wasn't necessarily the case.

In this book, I guide you to think about "alignment," like when puzzle pieces fit together perfectly to create a **total** picture of wellness. In order to achieve this level of balance, we need to look at not only the food on our plate, but the food off of our plate. Joshua Rosenthal, who is the founder of The Institute for Integrative Nutrition (where I became a certified health coach), refers to this as our primary foods. He says that loving life, having meaningful careers and embracing the things that feed us on a mental, emotional, psychological and spiritual level are even more important than the foods we eat.

Many people in our society are out of balance with total wellness because we're so fast-paced and since everything is amplified on social media, we often feel a few steps behind everyone else. So, we keep pushing ourselves harder and harder, which leads us to be out of alignment with our health. It is far too common to hear about people trying to improve their health by eating healthier and heading to the gym, but at the same time their marriages are falling apart or they're working at a job that has them feeling depleted – taking even more of a toll on their health.

Practicing healthy alignment sometimes means making tough decisions because maybe you've spiritually grown and evolved. Then, you might realize things that once suited you aren't in line with what you value now. When you're in alignment, life FEELS GOOD. You don't feel like you're on this busy, hamster wheel of life "doing, doing, doing" but rather you feel more in flow and balanced—therefore in a state of 'being," which allows you to feel more present with the joys of life. I like to say that alignment feels like being healthy **from the inside out.**

When you think about what it's like to feel healthy, your emotions even play a role, as you'll see more in Chapter 2. For me, getting onboard with this concept is about learning to "let go" of any expectations. And instead, setting goals - but allowing myself to "be okay" with the outcome if I didn't reach them (pertaining to business or ANYTHING else for that matter).

For sure, this shift in how I think about success and healthiness was a process for me and not a change I made in one day. When I look back, my life was definitely chaotic, and I always felt like something was off, but I could never put my finger on why that was happening. I know this to be true because when I became successful, I felt like "the angry achiever." This made no sense to me and I thought to myself, *I got to the top of the ladder; I'm making great money...where's my happiness?* I later learned that I was placing a high degree of pressure on myself to *control* the results I was always trying to achieve. This is obviously an unrealistic goal because there's never a guarantee. As a result, I was constantly beating myself up when I wasn't reaching those standards – which left me feeling very angry and frustrated.

Learning to "let go" of expectations and instead appreciate how far I've come by celebrating the little wins – has allowed me to look at the same situations with a different lens. This helped me find happiness again. In this book, chapter by chapter, I'm going to help you do the same things.

HOW TO USE THIS BOOK

Each chapter adds a protective layer to your well-being. The more things you're doing from this list - the stronger and healthier you'll be. Each component builds up your immune system - therefore, taking any stressors that weaken your immune system away. I've learned that our immune system is our ALLY & best friend - as it's always working to our advantage and defending us against foreign invaders, such as viruses and bacteria. When we take away stress, we take away DIS-EASE!

As I share my stories, you'll notice how a lot of the ideas are interconnected, all the way from Food to Detox and everything in between. This is because your body stores your thoughts and feelings and emotions, good and bad, right along with what you put into your body and how you take care of your needs. When you're not properly eating well, sleeping regularly, taking care of yourself, enjoying what you do, and who you're around and what's in your environment—the effects can be detrimental to your overall health and wellbeing. Fortunately, with the right information, you can address all these issues and feel better, as well as be more successful at what matters most to you.

Here's what we're going to cover:

Emotions: Our thoughts translate into feelings, and feelings impact our physical body. The good news is we can take charge of them and decide how we want to feel, no matter what outside circumstances are going on.

Food: Food is the fuel for our body. What we eat directly impacts how we feel. Eating sugar and processed food, translates into less energy. Whereas, eating living food such as colourful fruits and vegetables, will leave one feeling alive and vibrant. It's simple when you think about it, but profound when you apply it to every meal.

Sleep: Everyone is different, so if you're getting less sleep than you need, you'll feel the effects the next day. You know best what amount of sleep you need. Many people are so accustomed to being tired that they didn't even know how much more productive and well-rested they could feel.

Self-Care: This replenishes your energy. If you're constantly working, it's important to take breaks and prioritize yourself. When you do something fun or that brings you joy, you bring yourself into balance between work and play. It may feel weird at first to take this time for yourself, but when you get used to it, you'll see how much better you feel and that you get even more done.

Purpose: With a sense of purpose, you're excited to start the day and feel lit up inside. At a 9-5 job, many people feel drained and unfulfilled. They're thrilled to just have a day off. Having a sense of purpose makes us feel like we could work all day because we love what we're doing and it's in alignment with what we value most.

Detox: We live in a toxic world, and a lot of toxins are invisible. We don't even know how many are entering our body everyday because they're present in our environments. Fortunately, we can detox to get them out of our body and make changes to decrease the amount of toxins we're exposed to.

I'll tell you fun, personal stories along the way and let you know where to find more information if you want to go deeper on any of these topics. Most of all, be kind to yourself when you see me telling you something I used to do, and you might think, "that's totally me!" Just because right now that's where you are, you can change like I did.

Every step I took and every mindset I had to change is laid out for you as clearly as possible so you can hit the ground running and not spend years taking classes, reading books, and attending workshops like I did. Also, you don't have to go in order. For me, I was often working on more than one step at the same time, and sometimes I go back to a step when I realize there's still something I need to work on in that area of myself. So, start with the chapter that resonates with you the most and work through the steps in a way that makes the most sense for what you want to address most right now.

Do you like PRESENTS? Me, too! I created a free Self-Care Habits to Inspire Love and Joy Guide just for you, so pause right now and get it at www.deborahlobart.com/Self-Care. You deserve to start your healing journey today, one change at a time.

Making simple changes takes courage and isn't always easy, but it is always worth it. Your healthy lifestyle begins on the next page.

What if life was not happening to you, it was happening for you?

- Tony Robbins

CHAPTER 1

....

My Story

Before we dive into the steps of a healthy lifestyle, I want to share why I discovered this entire world of alternative medicine and how my professional/business and health pathway have always been intertwined. I just didn't always know that or understand how being healthier could also make me more successful and happier.

When I was 30 years old, I reached a plateau in my career and knew I needed a change. I was tired of working at jobs I didn't like. And I hated having others tell me what to do. I would often quit a job the second I was sick of it. For the most part, I couldn't keep a job for longer then 6 months. If I stayed at a job for longer then a year, that was a big deal for me, and I felt proud. I thought maybe there was something wrong with me. I didn't understand why I couldn't just settle. I mean, why couldn't I just find that "one thing" that I loved doing like everyone else? I job hopped quite a bit and life felt hard. Debt was piling up and I was tired of feeling worried about how I was going to pay my bills. Growing up I was led to believe that if I just worked hard and made a lot of money, that that was going to be the solution to everything and I would be successful, fulfilled and "live happily ever after."

Well, that wasn't necessarily the case.

In 2002, when I had just graduated from University with a degree in Psychology, I had a nice big loan to pay back of 20 grand. And as a matter of fact, when I graduated with this "degree" that everyone was preaching I "should" have, not only was it impossible to find a job, but now I had to figure out how I was going to pay back all the money that I borrowed.

To make ends meet, I started working as a sales manager at a popular health club around the corner from my house. Surprisingly, the pay was pretty good, and I actually had tons of fun working there. I enjoyed the people, the atmosphere and I thoroughly enjoyed working in a health and wellness space, but for some reason – it was ingrained in my mind that it wasn't "appropriate." Maybe it could work for a short time, but the long-term? It didn't have the fancy title and I learned that something more prestigious that looked good on paper was more important. Not to mention, I didn't need a university degree to get into this line of work.

As time went on, I ended up leaving the health and wellness industry and took a job at an advertising agency. I was paid $20,000 as a base salary and the rest I could earn in commissions. The money was decent but what really attracted me was the freedom of working from home and not having a boss breathing down my neck. I worked that job until my daughter Gabriella was born & started to get anxious thinking of the day I'd have to return. I really wanted to branch off and start my own business, but the thought of being self employed and running a 'traditional business' would again take away precious time from being with my daughter. I was at a loss. I was trying to figure out the solution but had no one to guide me. I would constantly be thinking of how I could earn a good income on my own terms, without sacrificing time away from my family? Was that even possible?

Then something interesting happened...

About 8 months into my maternity leave I was presented with an opportunity that was about to change everything for me – Network Marketing! I knew there were a lot of misconceptions about the industry, but I also knew that it was a legitimate business model - and with hard work, determination and daily consistent action, that it could be my ticket to freedom. So, without thinking twice, I trusted my intuition, jumped in and never looked back!

I started dreaming about the possibilities.

What if I never have to wake up to an alarm clock again and take long dreadful commutes? Yet, instead wake up ANYTIME of the day feeling *excited* to design my schedule the way "I" wanted to – instead of going to a job I hate?

What if I can work until 12 noon and then spend the rest of my day at my favourite park with my daughter and not have to ask a boss for permission?

What if I can own my dream home and book a spontaneous vacation to Italy without living paycheck to paycheck anymore?

Being able to do things I was never able to do, excite me to no end! It kept me up to all hours of the night.

This is where my real journey began.

I was so determined to succeed! I literally picked up every book on network marketing I could get my hands on. And started listening to CD's in my car at every opportunity I could. Momentum was picking up in my business as my schedule started getting busier and busier. The more people I shared the opportunity with, the bigger my business grew.

My first year in Network Marketing was a horrifying experience though. I only made a measly $3000 the entire year! My husband was questioning why I was still continuing and when I took my paperwork to my accountant's office, he laughed at me. He told me he's never seen anyone make any money in this industry. Although it was hurtful, I didn't care. I used it as fuel to get me motivated. I was relentless. No one was going to steal my dream or tell me that what I was after was not possible.

So, I continued working hard. At the end of my second year I reached a milestone and I was now making a full-time salary, exceeding what I made at any previous job I worked at. Life felt REALLY good. I was reaping the rewards of a wildly successful business and money was no longer an issue in my life. I was able to travel at a moments notice, drive a fancy car, move into my dream home and I was finally able to have the freedom of designing my own schedule the way I've always dreamt of. Being my own boss was something I always envisioned and now this was my reality. Things were going great!

Until life took a turn and my world flipped upside down.

It was the start of fall in October 2015 and I was heading out to the health food store to grab some snacks for a few guests that were coming over later in the day, when all of a sudden I was taken over by this dizzy spell, while I was walking down the aisle of the grocery store. I felt completely out of it like I was about to collapse. My vision was blurry, and I felt weak. I kept rubbing my eyes thinking something was wrong with them. It was odd because I never experienced anything like this before.

So not quite sure what was happening, I just hurried up what I was doing, grabbed my grocery's and got out of there as quickly as I could.

I thought maybe this was just a *temporary* thing and that I would sleep it off and have it gone the next day. But when the next day came and I was getting my kids ready for school, I noticed the symptoms again. It wasn't so obvious when I was in my home, but as soon as I left to take my son to preschool, I was taken back by the fluorescent lights in the hallway. They were so bright that it was bothering my eyes. I felt overwhelmed by it, that everything around me felt like it was appearing in slow motion.

From the conversations I was having with random parents and teachers, to just walking around the crowded hallways – I felt dazed and confused, like I was in some really bad dream – distorted from reality. I felt odd. And all I could think about was *I don't have time for this!* I'm too busy. I have a business to run and I need my brain to function. I was terrified and started developing anxiety – something I never experienced before.

The symptoms kept piling up from one month to the next, and I went from being a healthy, successful mom to dealing with chronic fatigue, brain fog, dizziness, nausea, depersonalization, chest pain, breathlessness, panic attacks, jumpy vision, light sensitivity, insomnia, headaches, hair loss, cysts, eczema, puffy eyelids and joint pain.

What was happening to me? I thought. I had huge responsibilities going on and I was at a loss because these symptoms popped up out of nowhere. None of them made logical sense to me. I was at a point in my life where I had an amazing and supportive husband, two beautiful small children, a healthy body and a thriving home-based business. In fact, I was the "happiest" I had ever been – or so I *thought*.

And so, the research began.

I started turning to various medical doctors, naturopaths, healers and coaches, to get advice. It was all so mysterious to me and I was desperately looking for answers to get better. As I looked for ways to heal, I began to document my journey. Unfortunately, it wasn't an easy journey. I not only spent three and a half years (amongst thousands of dollars) trying to figure it all out, but I went through A LOT of heartache. I was faced with tons of sleepless nights and many tough decisions to make. But I was determined to get to the bottom of things, so I could put this to rest and finally get on with my life.

Through all of my research I was realizing that living a healthy lifestyle was something I wasn't fully embodying. There was *so much more* that I was missing. It was about nourishing myself from the **inside out**. Looking at things holistically and considering the *mind, body* and *soul*. It was about walking away from things that no longer served me, digging deep, peeling off the layers and creating a meaningful life.

I hope my story inspires you and makes a difference in some powerful way.

Now, let's start your journey with a look inward for what may be going on with the mind that could be affecting how you feel.

Maybe the journey isn't so much about becoming anything. Maybe it's about unbecoming everything that isn't really you, so you can be who you were meant to be in the first place.

- Paul Coelho

CHAPTER 2

· ·

Emotions

When I reflect on what my life was like before these sudden symptoms appeared, I thought about my journey to success. And I remembered something - I was feeling pretty *blah* and wasn't quite sure how to snap out of it. Basically, I felt like I was in this constant fog, and there was an invisible wall between me and everyone around me.

I'd see people that had tons of energy and were happy all the time, and they started to annoy me. *How are these people always happy?* But I did my best to keep it together and put a smile on my face, pretending all was good in my life, but emotionally, I felt stressed.

Turns out, many of these emotions stemmed from thoughts I had at my first business conference in Las Vegas. I had been blown away--mostly in a good way, but also blown out of my comfort zone. I saw top earners in my company share their success stories on stage, and I thought, "there's no way I'm doing public speaking like them, EVER!" It was my number one fear! So, the fears I had around public speaking were present from day one of my business, and that was a tension I had to tackle to be in alignment with what I wanted, which was to be a top producer and earn a spot on that very stage.

The fear of my life staying the "same" was far greater than my fear of stepping into the spotlight. The problem was that I HATED the thought of public speaking so much and so anytime I had to do it, it was causing me enormous amounts of tension (the night before and all day leading up to the event). I would get so nervous that by the time I would show up to the venue, I felt drained - taking a toll on not only my health, but my happiness.

As I learned about fear, I discovered that it was coming from beliefs that had no basis in logic or the real world. It was incredibly freeing to look at my limiting beliefs that way because if they *weren't true*, there was no reason they should have any power over me. I started changing those beliefs to their opposites, like "I love speaking to an audience," "I'm so excited to change lives," "I will remember everything I need to say because I speak from my heart." This helped tremendously, creating a positive shift. But the changes I made didn't end there.

I noticed that I had tons more limiting beliefs in all kinds of areas in my life that were impacting my emotions, beyond just fear. I started paying closer attention to where else in my life that my emotions were holding me back. Here are some things I noticed and what I did about them:

- When I felt **tired and drained**, it was when I was surrounding myself with those who were complainers or spoke negatively (also known as, "energy vampires"). Naturally, this behaviour started to rub off on me. So, instead of agreeing with them and piling on my two cents, I consciously started to politely excuse myself from these negative conversations or I'd add a positive spin and change the topic. This way, I would leave conversations feeling good instead of drained.
- Anytime I would feel **frustrated and angry**, I noticed it was stemming from the false belief that "If I didn't reach my goals, I've failed." Instead of seeing the truth that I succeeded any time I learned something or gave my 100% to the task at hand. There was no reason to feel angry

or frustrated, so those feelings melted away. I started telling myself, "when I give 100%, I am always succeeding because I do my best."

- Anytime I would feel **sadness** pop up, I noticed it was because I was saying "yes" to things I didn't really want to do. So, I started to become honest with myself and began politely refusing to do things I wasn't interested in. I took "should" out of my vocabulary and only said "yes" to things I felt energized by.

You can control your emotions by prioritizing how you want to feel and embracing authenticity. I worked on this with a life coach who helped me remember to never lose the core of who I am or else, I'd never feel fulfilled.

LESSONS LEARNED

As a leader, I realized how much pressure I was putting on myself to perform PERFECTLY. I had this "made up story" in my mind that once I became successful, I needed to "have it all together." Truthfully, most people don't have it all together, even the successful ones. They just don't worry about it as much and instead focus on their purpose and positive thoughts. PLUS, having high standards of being "perfect" is simply unrealistic and is the LOWEST standard one could set for themselves, because there's no such thing as "perfect."

Another big aha was I thought I had to be "all professional," instead of "being me" - the one that likes to crack jokes and be silly! I learned that the opposite is true. Audiences connect more and prefer speakers that seem like someone they could relate to. Someone conversational and funny. Wow. Instead of trying to turn myself into someone I was not, it would serve me and my business better to just be real. I learned that the best speakers are authentic!

I learned that these were all *limiting beliefs* that were simply **not true**. Why? Because they weren't facts—I simply made these stories up in my head. They just prevented me from reaching my highest potential because I was stuck in "comparison mode" – these thoughts contributed to living with fear, doubt and lost passion.

Another thing I did is remind myself to b-r-e-a-t-h-e! Oxygen has positive effects on our nervous system. It's commonly known to reduce inflammation, lowers blood pressure and keeps stress at bay. I became conscious of how I was breathing, so instead of using my chest to breath in and out, I was concentrated on using my diaphragm instead – that really helps get me centered and balanced when I start to feel anxious. Did you know that you can't be anxious and breathe long slow exhalations at the same time? Learning to breathe correctly helped me manage my emotions on those tough days.

By opening myself up and being honest with how I was feeling was the key to my next stage of growth. Because suppressing all of that internally was taking a huge toll on my happiness.

Once I got clear on how I wanted to feel, which was happy and empowered, I helped myself and my team get on that path by being more of a leader than a manager for them. Here's the difference: a manager is someone that manages and asks for numbers and quotas. But a leader is different. A leader is someone that lights a fire inside them so they want it for themselves and believe they can achieve it.

HEALTHY LIFESTYLE ALIGNMENT

As I really examined my purpose, I saw that I wanted a great lifestyle and to make a difference in other people's lives, especially other moms like myself trying to do it all, all the time. I couldn't do that when I was weighed down by baggage of negative emotions that came from limiting beliefs. I felt empowered to change my life by getting off the hamster wheel of these limiting beliefs and embracing the truth. I no longer believed that I was "stuck" feeling the way I was feeling and that I could get myself in a peak state anytime I chose to. Knowing that I get to choose how I feel each and everyday in and out of work, is incredibly empowering.

Here are some things I do to keep my beliefs and emotions positive:

- Any time I want to feel **healthy and vibrant,** I turn on music and dance to an upbeat song or drink a nutritious smoothie or meditate. These activities help me feel balanced, centered, and powerful.
- To feel **love and warmth,** I show affection to my husband and children or focus on how I can help others. When I enhance how others feel, I feel better, too.
- When I want to be **fun and playful,** I'm silly with my kids when I can. And if I notice someone is angry or upset, I try to make a joke to lighten the mood. When we have a laugh, the other person instantly feels better, and I do, too.

The bottom line is that suffering is a **choice**! What we focus on expands. We can focus on being hard on ourselves or we can focus on being kinder and embrace self-love.

EXERCISE

1. Identify a limiting belief that you may have placed on yourself that is producing a negative emotion in your life.

2. What negative consequences have been happening in your life as a result of this?

3. What is the new story that you will be committing to going forward so that you can live in alignment with the core of who you *truly* are?

Is this going to cleanse
or clog me?

- Tony Robbins

CHAPTER 3

....

Food

If there was one complaint that I had growing up – it was that I ALWAYS felt bloated.

I almost forgot what it felt like *not* to be bloated because I felt like this all the time. I was skinny, but I always had this heavy feeling. I didn't look at belly bloat as a 'symptom' that needed to be addressed by a doctor though. And I also never associated any particular foods that I was eating that could have contributed to me feeling uncomfortable. It never dawned on me that maybe there was a correlation. Isn't that often how it is when you have an undiagnosed condition that's been there for so long, you don't even realize it's a problem?

Bloating was just a tip of the iceberg on what wasn't right with my health.

Although I had less time to prep healthy meals, I never thought my diet was ever "bad." The *worst* it would get at times would be meeting a co-worker at a coffee shop and ordering a cappuccino topped with cinnamon alongside a plain croissant. But then the croissant did start to become a regular breakfast routine as my schedule filled up with meetings. And the days if I was working from home, I would drive out of the house in my pjs and quickly grab a whole wheat bagel with eggs and a coffee. And to satisfy my sugar craving, I would grab two chocolate Timbits. I mean, what's two Timbits, right? So overall, things weren't *too* bad.

Then something shifted.

The dizzy spell I wrote about in Chapter 1 was the wake-up call. My medical doctor told me I was perfectly healthy, but that's not how I felt. It took all my energy just to get my kids off to school and accomplish simple tasks around the house. The first thing that came to mind was, "it must be something I'm eating" – I mean what else could it be, right? And while I was digging for answers to my questions about nutrition and what a truly healthy diet is, I found a retreat about living your healthiest life held in Fort Lauderdale, Florida. I thought, *perfect this will give me a much-needed getaway to the sunshine state, while maybe learning a thing or two about how to feel better.*

On the first day of the four-day retreat, one of the speakers led us in an exercise that stopped me dead in my tracks.

"Take out a sheet of paper and write down everything you ate in the last 24 hours," she instructed, so I did.

As I made my list, I felt pretty good about it and thought my food choices had been fairly healthy. That's why I was so confused why I felt so bad.

This was my list:

Grapes
Banana
Cheese
Crackers
Protein bar
Omelette
Toast
Almonds.

I mean that looks pretty healthy, right? I thought so! I got some protein in there. Some *whole wheat* bread and fruit, too. I hadn't eaten anything I'd call "junk food."

"Okay," she continued after a few minutes. "For each of the food items you listed, how many of them are water-rich?"

I reflected, *Hmm...maybe 20%?* Was that bad? The grapes and bananas had to count. With my number in mind, I looked up at the speaker.

"If you didn't say at least 70% of the foods you ate yesterday were water-rich, guess what? You're clogging up your body. You need at least 70% of your food to be water-rich so your body can cleanse itself."

Wow! This was a huge wake up call. I realized that vegetables were nowhere to be found in my diet. I also noticed that I was barely drinking any water. I could literally go days without water – which I knew wasn't healthy either. But I still did it because it wasn't affecting me 'in the moment.' Later on, I put the information together when I read more about the importance of water-rich foods in *Life-Changing Foods: Save Yourself and The Ones You Love With The Hidden Healing Powers of Fruits and Vegetables* by Anthony Williams, The Medical Medium. He says, "water that's inside fresh fruits and vegetables, herbs, and wild food possesses incredible healing qualities" (31). The more I thought about it, the more it made sense that hydration wasn't just about drinking water.

It was quite an adjustment when I started to introduce this new way of thinking about food and eating. I did an elimination diet so I could feel how different foods made me feel differently. So, for a month I eliminated the most-common foods that make people feel bad, including dairy, gluten, and processed sugars. All those foods can produce an inflammatory response, which includes guess what? Belly bloat. Check out Williams's book for more of an explanation of how those foods influence gut health.

I learned very fast during the elimination diet that I had a major sugar addiction. Here's how I knew I was addicted: any time I felt tired, I would reach for chocolate. Hello, Timbits. That's my weakness. I would have cravings for chocolate if I was tired and even drive to Baskin Robbins or Bulk Barn and grab chocolate to munch on. This habit was most pronounced when I was really tired. Now, for the first time, I realized that when I wasn't eating sugar, I wasn't having those times when I was extremely tired anymore. I had more energy—not less.

Something else amazing happened, too. My frequent headaches went away during my elimination month. At the end of the month, then, I would re-introduce one food at a time and see if I felt better, the same, or worse. I started to notice for the first time ever when I stayed off gluten and then began to eat even a small amount of it, I would get a headache within minutes. Sugar gave me instant fatigue. And where dairy is concerned, when I ate cheese or yogurt, I would feel bloated – this explains how I felt everyday after my morning cappuccinos. That feeling in my tummy was my body's way of communicating with me that these foods were not agreeing with me.

Depending on the food, my symptoms would vary. These are some of the ways my body would respond when I ate anything that contained processed sugar, dairy or gluten:

- low energy
- brain fog
- insomnia

- heart rate increase/decrease
- nausea
- headaches

All of these symptoms can be linked to inflammation. The good thing is that as Williams explains it, inflammation can be healed, and it doesn't even take that much time to start feeling better when you eat a healthier diet and make that part of your everyday habits.

Here are a few healthy diet changes I made and stick to them for my healthiest lifestyle:

1. Eat More Real Foods

I added more real, whole foods to my daily meals. This meant completely eliminating bread and dairy from my diet (as these were contributing to too many of my symptoms) and then replacing those foods with things like smoothies, soups, and salads. I committed to making sure my plate was at least 75% living foods. **If any food came in a box, wrapper or with an ingredient list I didn't understand - I wasn't eating it.** I wanted to eat whole foods that came from the earth, such as: fresh fruits and plenty of colourful vegetables – which is good news because the meals I was making more often were things I'd always enjoyed eating.

2. Go for Greens

I learned to love eating things like kale salads, brussels sprouts, broccoli and asparagus. There are some super delicious ways of seasoning these green veggies, so they are nice and tasty--or even throwing a handful of spinach in a smoothie is a great way to add more greens. So, 75% of my plate is greens because they neutralize excess acid in the body (Williams 146-7).

3. Say Goodbye to Sugar

In terms of sugar, I didn't realize that I was including so much of it in my diet. It was not only causing me to keep my clothes snug and not lose those extra pounds after pregnancy, but I felt bloated and not my best. Here's some great advice from Sarah Wilson, author of *I Quit Sugar: Your Complete 8-Week Detox Program and Cookbook* (2014) on sugar consumption: "the average woman should have no more than 24-36 grams of sugar per day (aside from fruit)." Doing this was a game changer for me in the *initial* stages of my healing journey.

This doesn't mean I never have sweet foods. The fruit I add to my breakfast is amazing and tastes way sweeter now that I'm not eating so much sugar all day. I often make a nutritious breakfast smoothie with filtered water, frozen strawberries, a banana and a dash of wild blueberry powder or some greens powder – depending on the day, because I switch things up, so I don't get bored.

4. Cut Caffeine

After having a cup of coffee almost every day of the week, I decided to see what life would be like if I completely eliminated it from my diet. Coffee is an acid. And from everything I was hearing from various experts, I came to my own conclusion that if it stimulates your heart rate to go up, affects your adrenals and puts wear and tear on my nervous system with all the stress I was under – I didn't want to add any more pressure. My adrenals were already burnt out and caffeine would further aggravate it.

Lesson Learned:

I had an epiphany – I always *thought* I ate healthy. I was shocked at the retreat in Florida when I learned that 'whole wheat' bread caused inflammation. I always believed "whole wheat" to be healthy--but where did this belief come from? I guess it was the years of marketing in the media that instilled this belief in me. I ate bread almost everyday. And I was bloated everyday, and everyday I always had stomach aches, felt groggy and got frequent headaches. But I had never put two and two together until I did my own research about having a truly healthy diet.

It's unbelievable how much conflicting information there is out there. And although there are so many different dietary theories like paleo, keto, vegetarian and so on – I really do believe that despite what one decides to follow, one thing remains consistent. **A diet rich in colourful living foods is essential to well-being**. There are too many essential nutrients that we'd be giving up otherwise and can't be found in a pill.

It's very easy to think you're doing everything right, only to be told later that it's not. For the longest time, I thought I needed to eat 'enough' protein – otherwise, I'd be low in energy. Or that for my genetic type, that Keto was ideal – so I'd be jumping from this theory to that. But at the end of the day, my body's the judge. And I knew that I was feeling great with more fresh fruits and vegetables.

The first 7-10 days of this switch, I'll admit – I was in fact feeling worse. I had major fatigue, even worse than before I started. But I remained patient and as I continued this new way of eating, I couldn't believe how fast the weight was falling off. I wasn't counting calories anymore. I wasn't counting grams of protein (there's protein in plants) - I was just focused on consuming a water rich diet with REAL foods. This meant shopping on the outside aisles of my local grocery store and purchasing organic produce to reduce toxic chemicals, as I'll speak to more in the Detox chapter.

HEALTHY LIFESTYLE ALIGNMENT

Eating too few whole foods was out of alignment with the life I wanted as the top-performing leader I wanted to be. Energy and mental clarity are crucial for this role; therefore, the more I stick to these new eating habits the better I was able to perform at work. And then this of course trickles down to being able to take care of my kids better in my daily activities as well. Another big shift I made to be a better mom and businesswoman is to work on my sleep. More about that in the next chapter.

EXERCISES

1. In the last 24 hours write down everything you have eaten or drank.

2. Look at your list - what percentage of your diet is made up of water-rich foods?

3. What are some foods that you love that have a high-water content?

4. What are some of your symptoms that you think can be addressed by changing your eating habits?

5. What aspects of your nutrition are you committing to change?

You can eat all the kale in the world but if your life is chaotic your health will be in jeopardy.

- Joshua Rosenthal

CHAPTER 4

Sleep

"I miss back when you would play with me," my daughter said. She had just come into my bedroom and was still in her pajamas, with tears streaming down her face.

My heart melted, and this was another huge wake-up call. As much as I didn't want to believe it was true - it was. Almost everyday, I was rushing to make dinner for her and my son, Bobby, so that I could scoot off to my next work meeting. A clear look of disappointment would spread across her face as I would say, "Mommy needs to leave now." Her eyes would gloss over, ready to burst into tears, and I'd feel so guilty. But I was so busy and consumed with work that everything else fell by the wayside. I was so busy, I barely had time to breathe.

I couldn't slow down no matter how hard I tried. Even if I took time to relax and play with the kids, my mind wouldn't be there. I'd be thinking "you could be getting so much done now!' I'd be mentally thinking of things I need to add to my (never ending) to-do list or my next big goal I had to accomplish. So, needless-to-say, my mind was on overdrive, and I didn't know how to shut the darn thing off. And it was costing me my relationship with my then-6 yrs. old daughter.

Even during my yoga classes, I'd go there to try and unwind - but even still, my mind would be racing. I'd think of errands to run, what I was going to make for dinner, phone calls to return and catching up on emails and texts. It's no wonder I felt depleted, even after a yoga class.

27

With my mind always on overdrive, this was also affecting my sleep. It was also at a time where I was at the height of my business and going for the next promotion. So, I was physically exhausted and drained but since it was a feeling, I was very accustomed to – I didn't think much of it. I did notice that I'd wake up with headaches and fogginess the less sleep I had, even though my eating habits improved.

Busy was an understatement. Ever since 2012 when my son was born, I hadn't been sleeping well. For years, I was dealing with chronic fatigue, but I just brushed it off as being a busy mom of two young children and having a successful business. But these are warning signs that need to be addressed early before they lead into bigger health challenges.

In 2015 I hired my first coach at the height of my business to help me take it to the next level. I was so nervous, though. I never worked with a coach before and had no idea what to expect. But I also knew that growth only happens out of my comfort zone so I went for it.

Here's what I recall of our first conversation:

"When I set this appointment, I wanted a coach to help me with my network marketing business to help me grow it to the next level," I said. "But unfortunately, I've been feeling super tired lately, to a point that I haven't been doing much. And I'm not sure why that is." I hoped she could still help me since my problem wasn't as clear to me as I had thought coming into the appointment.

She zeroed in right away to my adrenal fatigue diagnosis, which my doctor had told me and gave me a protocol for, and then that was it. She explained that adrenal fatigue is stress-related, which I knew, but then she explained what that meant.

"The deal is that we have adrenals that pump out cortisol that pumps us up, right? And that's great when you need it. We have a store house when we need it but what happens is when you're lacking energy – we draw on those supplies. Sound familiar?"

"Totally," I said. "If I always lack energy, then I keep drawing on my supplies to the point that I fatigue my adrenal glands?"

"Yes! You borrow energy from your adrenal bank. And then it goes into overdrive, and you aren't getting energy from anywhere else, other then artificially through coffee and sugar (or whatever other stimulants). If you have adrenal fatigue, you're probably craving coffee or sugar, right?"

"Yes! I'm working on that for my health."

"Okay, so that's all outside sources which are artificially fuelling you. Then, it's up to your adrenal glands to keep you on the go, go, go, go.... So, I bet you're probably feeling tired during the day and can't sleep at night."

"Ummm, I feel tired ALL the time!"

"Okay, so they're really low and working overtime. Give them a break."

"Ya," I said softly.

"In addition to diagnosing your adrenal fatigue, did they tell you what to do?"

"Ya, he gave me supplements."

"And?"

"The pills helped. It helped for about 4 months but then I wasn't totally taking them after 4 months, and then I guess it came back but it was milder and then I went back to the doctor..."

"Okay, so there's a little bit of a theme here Deborah. Umm, well it works when I'm doing the diet and I felt better but then, I stopped doing it and I stopped feeling better."

I started giggling, a bit embarrassed, as I was starting to realize the obvious.

"Look, the bottom line with adrenal fatigue is supplements are great and all, but really, it's **lifestyle!**"

"Uh huh," I said quietly as it slowly sunk in.

"Period. It's **lifestyle**," she said again. "You can only push yourself so much. And you're probably really good at pushing yourself but it's not working for you. Something has to change. The other thing is you need 'you' time."

"Ya, I go to the gym, I go for a massage – I do things for me, I do."

"Okay, so you said gym, massage. What else?" She asked. I told her about my mani-pedi and shopping trips, feeling pretty good about all the things I do for me.

"Awesome. Do you **sleep?**" She asked.

"Umm, not....no!" Wow, I couldn't even answer that question. Especially since my son was still sleeping in our bed, I really hadn't slept well in three years.

"Okay, so mani's and pedi's and shopping and all that kind of stuff is awesome and that's great but it's not really deeply for you. So, for example, for you would be something where you could shut off completely. Like the massage, is a great example. A bubble bath is also wonderful. The gym and exercise are still great, but quite frankly when you're in adrenal fatigue, you do not want to do cardio because that's worse. You want to do something gentle. Not cardio. You're making it worse that way."

She went on to tell me to get a good night's sleep every night and even take naps in the middle of the day. "THAT is doing 'for you' what you really need. The mani-pedis are great. But that's not going to fully replenish you like having the bed to yourself without a leg landing in your face."

I knew she was right. After all, he would flip around in his sleep like a sumo wrestler, and I had to keep one ear open to make sure I didn't roll over on him.

"I'm trying," I said. "My husband and I bought him a car bed because he really loves cars but he doesn't sleep in it so we told him we're going to sell it but we'll give him one more chance and if he doesn't, then we're going to get rid of it. But we haven't actually done that. This just happened within the last few days."

"Okay, so let me get this straight. His choice is to stay in the bed with you or stay in his new car bed."

"Yup, or we're going to get rid of it."

"Okay, so he's thinking 'alright, I'll just stay in your bed! I'm okay with that!'"

We both started cracking up. As I started to hear how ridiculous the whole thing sounded.

"Is there another strategy?" She asked. Maybe one that your intuition is telling you or that you heard of how to handle it?"

"Well it's hard to have a conversation with a 3-year old," I said.

"If you did, what would you say?" She asked.

"That mommy needs to sleep, with a laugh! Period." Next, she helped me come up with language I could share with him about how I need to sleep, and after all, he does care about how I feel and wouldn't want to be making me tired.

This was the first time I was realizing how much I was neglecting my own needs and how crappy I was feeling because of it. But grateful to have someone point out that I had more control over the situation then I was acknowledging.

LESSONS LEARNED

I went home and had the conversation with my son about sleeping in his own bed. He blinked at me with his cute, blue eyes, and it was hard for me to be firm, but I was. It took a little positive reinforcement, but in the end, he started choosing to sleep in his new, big bed like the big boy he wanted to be.

This change helped me be more present for both of my kids. Not being on the go all the time, gave me time back to be with my daughter. Same with my son, who's 8 years old now. We wrestle together, as it's one of his favourite things to do – "you can't catch me," he says – as his eyes light up. Then we race and try to catch each other around the room, as we both laugh hysterically. This is what life is about – the pleasure in the little things.

HEALTHY LIFESTYLE ALIGNMENT

Instead of a luxury, now I see that sleep is an essential component to living my healthiest lifestyle. If I don't go to bed at a normal time by 9:30 to fall asleep by 10, I get a second wind and then it takes longer to fall asleep. I wasn't used to downtime at first, and it felt strange prioritizing myself. Especially if you're a mom, you might have to adjust to it, too. I was so used to having a million things going on around me all at once. But this was an important clue to my recovery ~ *rest and relaxation.*

EXERCISE

Try one of the following ideas I've incorporated into my own sleep ritual and see which ones help you sleep. Each time you try another sleep ritual, journal about how you feel the next day and give it at least 7 days so you can keep track of what works better for you.

1. Limit technology before bed

Just like a computer needs to wind down, the brain needs to wind down too. Our brains are processing way more information than a generation ago. With the constant flow of emails, texts and social media hype, our minds get put into overdrive. Avoiding any work, cell and/or computer usage 2-3 hours before bed will help tremendously. *Tip: You may want to put your phone on airplane mode and keep it in another room to avoid any temptation*

Day 1:
Day 2:
Day 3:
Day 4:
Day 5:
Day 6:
Day 7:

2. Sleep in a dark room

Any bit of light suppresses melatonin (and high levels of melatonin is needed with "deep quality" sleep). So, you're going to want your room dark! If there's light streaming in from your shutters, you may want to invest in dark curtains. Or to make things simple, you can throw on a sleep mask.

Day 1:
Day 2:
Day 3:
Day 4:
Day 5:
Day 6:
Day 7:

3. Fasting

If your bedtime is at 10pm, stop eating by 7pm so your body has the 2-3 hours it needs to digest its food before lying down. This may sound tough if you're used to snacking. In which case, if absolutely needed – grab something super light, like a handful of fruit if you feel you need it.

Day 1:
Day 2:

Day 3:
Day 4:
Day 5:
Day 6:
Day 7:

4. Relax

There's nothing more relaxing than taking a hot bath before bed, in my opinion. This helps to unwind after a busy day & lowers the stress hormone cortisol. But if baths are not your thing, maybe taking a walk in nature or doing a gentle yoga class is? Choose what feels good to you.

Day 1:
Day 2:
Day 3:
Day 4:
Day 5:
Day 6:
Day 7:

I realize life gets busy and implementing all of these at the same time may be tough. But if you can slowly work your way up so that you're hitting each one of these, that's something to celebrate! Try keeping a journal to track your progress with how you're feeling. Slowly but surely if you keep at it, your sleep will improve, and you'll be feeling well rested again!

My life is joyously balanced
with work AND play.

- Louise Hay

CHAPTER 5

....

Self Care

As a successful network marketer, I was constantly on social media, answering questions and taking call after call. I was glued to my phone and social media. I didn't quite have any boundaries in place.

I had always worked this way, so I didn't know any other way to be successful. No matter how much I did, I felt it wasn't enough. I would work 10-hour days and anything not-work related felt like a waste of time. I was so focused on the 'achieving' and 'doing' and not enough time on the 'being.' Does this ever happen to you? Where your mind is always on overdrive thinking of the next thing and the next, to check off of your to-do list?

One of the biggest misconceptions we are led to believe by society is that a busy person is a successful person. This is a lie because a busy person fills their time with just about anything that's not productive, while a successful person is intentional.

For me personally, I noticed a trend. Anytime I focused on doing **too much**, I noticed my health declining. This went on for years until I learned the power of alignment. I learned that if I work more than 4 hours a day in front of my computer, I will start getting a headache and my symptoms would plop right back. Prior to finding this out, my family would find me at my computer all day long.

Checking things off my list made me happy (in the short-term) and so it was always my top priority. Because that list never ended, there was always something else that would magically appear. I was essentially aligned with being busy and hustling.

Then, with help like my coach from the previous chapter, I learned self-love and to put myself on my schedule. Before, I was always last on my list, and if I didn't have time, I wasn't on my calendar. I started putting myself on my list and will only be there for others when my own cup is full.

Our bodies aren't designed to always be working, so we're out of alignment with our health to be always hustling. To be in alignment with wellness, it's a matter of listening to your body and knowing when you're doing too much. I recognize the signs that it's time to take a break now. If I start to feel tired or my neck is sore, I need to take a break and, in many cases, I'll go for a walk.

Nowadays, if I work hours in front of the computer and take mini-breaks, I feel better. I stretch every 30 minutes to grab a glass of water. I might put on a song and have a dance party or take a personal phone call. I don't know how else I could have such a flexible lifestyle to take care of myself without my network marketing business where I can be my own boss – so, I'm very grateful!

The healthy boundaries I hold for myself help my team set healthy boundaries, too. You can balance work and play, because what's the point of working if you're not also enjoying pleasure? After all, network marketing is about duplication of a process, so if I model a lifestyle of burnout and sickness, that's what my team will replicate, and then they'll most likely quit. Instead, by being a role model for putting myself first, I show them how network marketing is part of a sustainable and healthy lifestyle.

I find that when I'm well-rested, I'm more creative and can get more done in four hours than I used to do in 10 hours. This is possible because in the 4-hour workday, I'm more laser-focused and at a higher vibration energetically because I'm in alignment with my healthy lifestyle that includes self-care.

My team members also get to learn to be independent leaders instead of having to rely on me for everything. Learning self-reliance empowers them to have more ownership of their businesses, which is also an important growth step.

One of the most profound shifts for me (and one I teach to my team) happened when I learned to divide my day up into two parts a) work and b) self love. This subtle change in my routine has made a massive impact on my overall health & happiness. Especially keeping in mind that one of the main reasons I've chosen to be an entrepreneur is the flexibility of being able to choose my own hours.

Here's what my day usually looks like:

A) Work (9:00 am – 1:00 pm)

I remember the first day that I worked for only four hours. I gave myself a limit and I was firm. I didn't work a minute longer. I would drop my kids off at school for 8:30 am, make my strawberry smoothie, then work from 9am to 1pm. And I was mindful to give myself a short 5-minute break every 30 minutes to stretch, take a walk or any other way that would give my body a break somehow.

At 1pm I was already feeling like a million bucks. Because now I had something to look forward to – FUN!

This is where part two of my day started.

B) Self Love (1:00 pm onwards)

So, by the time I was done with my "work for the day," I would reward myself with some me-time before having to pick up my kids from school. So that would leave me with about 3 hours to choose something from my self care list (which you can reference on my website)!

At first, it can be a struggle to give yourself permission to have fun, but once you get the hang of it, you'll have tons of self-love activities you enjoy. I've listed some of my personal favourites below:

Nature

I started to break my day up, taking short breaks throughout the day to get away from my office and get plenty of fresh air. I had never appreciated nature so much before. This did wonders for my spirit. I would come back home, take one look in the mirror and feel fresh and vibrant.

My body was craving nature and being in the fresh air and trees helped me get grounded. And when it was sunny, it was double the pleasure! The sun has healing powers, boosting serotonin, which is a 'feel good' chemical in the brain.

Exercise

Healing my body required plenty of movement. I can honestly say that yoga was one of the biggest things that helped me get my health back. It helped me lower my stress levels, breathe fully and get present. If you've ever been to a yoga class, you must have heard endless praise to take deep breaths. That's because the depth of our breath directly affects the state of our mind and the health of our body. Oxygen gives our body life and energy.

The point is choosing something enjoyable so I would stick with it and want to do it daily. Ideally, you'll want to do something active for 30 minutes each day. Movement is so important for mental health (as this is another way to increase serotonin). On the days I wasn't doing yoga, I was doing weight training at the gym or going for a walk. I also love to dance, which brings me so much joy. Back in the day, I never considered my workout a 'real' work out unless my heart was pounding. Recovering from adrenal fatigue, I have learned that I needed to tone it down and do lower impact, so I choose my workouts wisely.

Fun + Adventure

I remember one of my coaches asking me 'so what do you do for fun?' I had to really think long and hard about that one. I wasn't having fun anymore, although it was one of my deep-rooted values. When she gave me permission to start having fun again, it was like a fire was lit within me. I was reminded about something *so simple*, yet so profound—have fun. *Why wasn't I doing this?* The day I shifted my mindset to **allow** myself to work AND play, my whole world changed that instant. Spontaneity brought my passion back and I had greater balance already. So, I would use this time to choose whatever lit me up in the moment.

Brain Dump

This has helped me de-clutter my mind and restore balance on so many levels. Especially when I had several symptoms going on and things were a mystery as to why, recording my feelings, symptoms, what I ate and did each day helped bring clarity as to why certain things were happening. I wouldn't have noticed some patterns if it weren't for jotting them down (as sometimes I can't even remember what I ate for breakfast).

Also, doing a brain dump before bed helps me unwind and take things out of my head and onto paper for a more restful sleep. I could be writing down anything from business ideas that pop up, to what I love and appreciate about myself.

Meditate

Every morning I woke up and instead of reaching for my phone to let news and gossip fill my head, I splashed some water on my face, grabbed a nice cup of hot lemon water and started my morning meditation. A simple 5 minutes of morning mantras were enough to get my mindset set up on the right track so I can conquer the day ahead with positivity.

I especially find it helpful to do gratitude meditations, and this can be really quick. When things weren't going as planned, it was very easy to have this negative downwards spiral in my emotions. So, on my worst days, instead of complaining about what was going wrong, I would remind myself and take 3 seconds to choose gratitude.

Essential Oils

One of my favourite things that have become my new obsession is having my diffuser running all day – whether it be in my home or car. I have a sweet-smelling aroma to purify the air and get me into the mood of what I am craving most. If I want a little pick me up to lift my mood and be more focused and productive, I'll diffuse some wild orange and spearmint and if I want to unwind and calm down before bed, I'll diffuse some Frankincense or Vetiver.

I love that taking care of myself can include changes to my environment that help me feel better and also smell great.

LESSON LEARNED

SO, IMAGINE THIS....

I've gotten my most productive 4 hours of quality work out of the way, had some 'me' time, so when I'm ready to pick up my kids – I am in a great physical state. I am giving them the best of me instead of the rest of me and I have no other distractions. I keep my phone in a separate room from me in the house. My mind stops thinking about 'what I need to do next' for work & I'm officially 'unplugged' for the day. This allows me to feel present **with the people that matter most**. No more scatterbrain with my to-do lists going on in my head while I'm with my kids or having my son tell me to stop looking at my phone when he's trying to talk to me.

To give you an idea, by 4pm the only thing I have on my mind is family. It's such a great feeling because when I'm on my way to the bus stop to pick them up after school, I'm so *excited* to see them and find out how their day was. I feel so *connected* and *present* in the moment. Once we're at home, I start preparing dinner. Now this is where another shift has happened for me. I used to HATE cooking. I looked at this as another chore. Having very little time in my busy life, I felt like ordering out every night to save me the time and clean up. But then I dealt with the guilt of feeling like I'm not being the best mom by giving them the healthiest meals.

But our mindset is powerful.

It's very hard to enjoy cooking when I have that belief that I hate it. But the good news is that – I can *change* my thoughts. Which changes my beliefs. And so that's what I did.

If eating a healthy meal is part of self care and it's also something we do when we're with people we love, then I'm going to start looking at cooking as part of self care time necessary to nourish myself and my family's body.

How's that for changing my perception?

This has been **profound** for me. Because as busy as I am, health is my number one priority, therefore, home cooking is right up there. This is how I have *chosen* to reprogram my mind.

Another shift has been getting my kids involved in the kitchen too. So now I get to bond with them. And they're learning about healthy food. It's so cute. Bobby's only 8 years old, & he LOVES making his own salads. He mixes the arugula and romaine lettuce in a bowl with the dressing. He'll be the one to sprinkle salt and pepper & I'll add in the lemon juice and olive oil.

Gabriella's a huge help too – she's 11 and LOVES doing things around the kitchen (even the dishes – yay)! But what I love is that she gets a healthy amount of fruits and vegetables into her diet because she helps me peel, cut and wash a variety of them. Because she's involved in the process, she enjoys eating them more. She's already planning her own cooking channel.

HEALTHY LIFESTYLE ALIGNMENT

I used to jeopardize my health by working too much. What's wealth without health? You can do even greater work and be financially successful when you're aligned with a healthy lifestyle.

In the beginning, my definition of success was very different. I thought to be successful and happy, I would need a lot of money to buy anything and travel anywhere. Now, I think success is about a balanced lifestyle, so you need enough money to live a healthy lifestyle, but it also means enjoying quality time with loved ones.

You can have it all, as long as you're in balance between money, health, and happiness. Stuff is just one piece of the puzzle to becoming truly happy. Being conscious of how you're living every day brings you into alignment.

REFLECTION QUESTIONS

Did you get my FREE Self-Care Habits to Inspire Love and Joy Guide? If not, grab it at www.deborahlobart.com/Self-Care. Then, we're going to create your own with the exercise below.

1. Write a list of how you want to feel each day. For example, inspired, energized, peaceful, fulfilled, amused, healthy....

2. Write a list of the things you can do each day that will make you feel this way. Maybe these are things you can do before you start work or during a lunch break. Take your time with this one & enjoy it!

What if enjoying your life became
your greatest achievement?

- Tony Robbins

CHAPTER 6

· ·

Purpose

As my journey was unfolding, I was beginning to realize that my goal for creating this *big life* when I was a kid stemmed from thinking that material things would make me happy. When I was 9 years old, I got to do dance lessons for one year, but then couldn't continue. We took road trips, but we weren't able to take major vacations my friends took. I had a great childhood, but I dreamt of being able to afford whatever I wanted to do. My parents called me a dreamer, and I dreamt of having a lot of money and not having to worry about it. I believed that if money gave me freedom I would live happily ever after.

However, as an adult I see that's clearly not the case. Don't get me wrong, freedom is still very much a huge value of mine - but even with my successful network marketing business and the freedom money can buy, something was still *missing*. I had achieved a great life - the nice house, a fancy car, a wonderful family and so on - I was very appreciative of all of these things. I booked spontaneous spa getaways with my mom, and we'd get our hair and nails done, or I'd go shopping with my mom and letting her pick out whatever she wanted to buy. I would also book a spontaneous trip to self-help and personal development events with Tony Robbins, Robin Sharma, Jack Canfield—some of which included hotels that cost amounts that would normally be out of reach to me.

I was content, but my soul was yearning for more. I didn't know what was still wrong since I was financially successful. I didn't want to feel like I was just going through the motions so I started taking a lot of personal development courses I hoped would help me get to the next rank in my business.

I wanted something deeper, and I know now that what I was looking for is a purpose, to enjoy what I do and why instead of achieving milestones. My search for purpose made me open to ideas I would've normally ignored and thought a little weird. Then...things started to strangely line up. It's like the universe conspires to send you little messages at the *right* time because you're **open** to receiving them.

It happened to me when a random email landed in my inbox. It was perfect timing. It was the *catalyst* that was about to start a whole new chapter for me - & one that would contribute significantly to my healing journey (although, I had no idea at the time). It was a free 15-minute psychic offering. And I was really curious to see what this was all about because not only was she a psychic, but also a business coach.

So, I hopped on a Skype call with her - Amber was her name. And I felt connected to her immediately. I loved her energy. She was so vibrant. And kind. And down to earth. And I had this inner knowing that she was about to give me some really great insight. The call started off at a quick pace.

"Do you mind if we dive right into this call, because we only have about 15 minutes and I have a lot to share with you.

"Absolutely! Please go ahead," I said.

"Well, this career of yours has been keeping you from reaching your highest potential. It's been great for the last decade and it's been that gateway for you to be a platform and a step into exploring something else," she explained.

"Really? Hmm, but I poured my heart and soul into it," I said.

"Yes, you've actually been restless for quite some time. And it's when you're curious & start to explore, that you start to find out what you're *truly passionate about* & when we find out what we're passionate about, that's how we find our calling."

"You have a gift, Deborah. You're a leader and the world needs to hear your story. Your soul has been craving more for a while. You have so much more to offer. You just need to trust the process and have faith."

"Hear my story? What story do people need to hear from me?" I was confused when I got off the call. But I kept thinking about our conversation over and over again because for whatever reason - she got me excited, and I was FEELING alive again (something I hadn't felt in a while).

But the more I thought about it the more it made sense - I felt like I was doing the same thing every day, day in and day out. My daily tasks were robotic, and I'd lost touch with how I was feeling everyday - instead of tuning into my true self and listening to my heart.

Coincidentally, hours after our call I was in my kitchen making lunch and I had a business podcast playing in the background with someone interviewing Alexi Panos, who is an entrepreneur and motivational speaker. Everything she said really resonated with me. It got to a point where during the interview she said something that stopped me right in the middle of what I was doing, so I could grab a pen and paper and jot it down.

"When you're not living in your *soul*, you're going to constantly be feeling that you're searching for something you don't have the answer to. And the answer is you."

Wow. Something clicked.

When I was building my network marketing business - I was so wrapped up in the doing and the achieving, that I was forgetting the most important part. Enjoying the journey. Finding joy. So, I was at a point where I was ready to start peeling back the layers and doing more of what lights me up. And in order to do more of that, I needed to reconnect with the core of my being and follow my passions.

"Success without fulfillment is the ultimate failure" ~ Tony Robbins

So, without hesitation I hired a designer, launched a website and started a blog. After all, I had spent thousands upon thousands of dollars during my personal development and health journey that I felt I had so much to share. I started sharing snippets of what I had learned on social media and blog posts. I started going more public and allowing people into my life.

I once read that "the risk I'm afraid of taking could be the one that changes another's life!" I believe this is really true. It's so easy to brush off things that I've learned as insignificant, but we really never know who needs to hear that message.

This started to spark something in me and all I could think about was writing and teaching and making a difference - in whatever way I could - books, blogs, courses. I felt lit up inside - something I hadn't felt in a very long time!

Lesson Learned

Doing something that I love, that lights me up and gets me up in the morning is DOING something 'for' my health - because it doesn't feel like work and does something positive for my body. Then, I chose to take time off from building my business and focus on going back to school and learning about health and blogging. It feels so good to feel successful because I'm happy, not because I'm meeting arbitrary goals.

Sometimes making those tough decisions are the best ones and our biggest lessons. I didn't understand this at the time because I was still "in" it and I felt torn making the decision. Guilt was creeping in when I thought about taking time for myself. But I didn't have a choice. I knew that in order to regain my health, I needed to pay attention to what 'felt' good. That meant honouring my feelings and taking a break from business. Thankfully, I built a residual income and that didn't mean I had to resign - it just meant, I needed to take some time for me to reflect and be okay with taking a break from the hustle.

For the very first time - I listened to myself, and it felt soooo good!

I checked back in with Amber and told her how I was doing. This was what she said:

"It's tough for you to see this right now, but I promise you – this moment will be your biggest lesson. I don't believe there are wrong choices. There are choices with harder consequences and choices with easier consequences. You feel guilty because you feel like you 'should' have done something other than what you did. But in actuality, you did the best thing possible. Something that I have a feeling you will teach and guide others to do.

Which is honoring yourself first. That is always doing the right thing. **You're allowing yourself to be honest & true to you**. Something you've avoided for a while. You needed this. It wasn't serving you. You knew that. The question was always whether or not we could seamlessly transition you from this home-based business to something else to honour those you've brought on under you. But sometimes things can't be 'perfect' or 'seamless' especially if it's hurting you as much as it is. You have really good instincts. I want you to continue to trust and honour those. You have so much more to give and that side of you is awakening even stronger!"

I loved her response and felt comforted. I was also reminded of this quote that I'll leave you with:

The things you are passionate about are not random, they are your calling – Fabienne Fredrickson

HEALTHY LIFESTYLE ALIGNMENT

Amber put me on a path to see that there was more to life, so I went to health coaching school. I saw that I wasn't fully in alignment with how I was running my business and doing everything offline. I wanted to support my team to do more than only sell products. I want us to all live our best lives, and align health, wealth and happiness.

Reflection Questions

1. What are you passionate about?

    Many people spend their whole lives seeking their purpose, but our purpose is to be in joy. Think about your childhood and what you loved doing before all of your responsibilities came into your life. What could you do for hours that feel like minutes? Make a list of these things and try implementing one or two of them going forward.

2. Contribution

    Finding a way to help others can add so much joy to our lives - whether it's our kids, our spouse, our colleagues, our friends. When you look at the people in your life, they surround themselves around you because you touch them in some way. What is it that people love about you? How can you make a difference in your own unique way?

The root cause of nearly all disease -- cancer, diabetes, heart disease, it doesn't matter - is an overload of toxins and chemicals accumulating inside your body. Period.

- Ty Bollinger

CHAPTER 7

• •

Detox

The alarm went off one morning at 7 a.m. with the intention to go to the gym. But I was really pushing myself to go, as I didn't have the energy. I had prepped my gym clothes the night before to make things easier, but I felt like a zombie as I put on my LuluLemons. My mind was thinking, *how effective is my workout really going to be?* I could barely keep my eyes open. But despite how I was feeling, I ignored it because I was getting frustrated with myself that I wasn't working out as often. I used to be a gym rat, working out 6 days a week. The gym was a passion and kept me sane.

So, I went to the gym. I had my boots and winter jacked on so when I arrived, I had to go straight to the change room to change into my running shoes and put my jacket and boots into the locker. When I was walking out of the changing room and heading to the weight room, I felt disoriented and confused on where to exit. By this point, I was having strange neurological symptoms such as depersonalization that was terrifying me.

Although I was taking many steps to live a healthier lifestyle - I knew there was still something **deeper** that was going on that *still* needed to be addressed. But doctors weren't helping, and I was tired of chasing my tail - going from doctor to doctor for answers and feeling like this was being turned around on me--as if this was a 'mental' thing and not a 'physical' one. It made no sense. How could it be all in my head that I felt so disoriented with debilitating fatigue?

Finally, a few days later, I was driving home from the grocery store and suddenly felt shortness of breath/difficulty breathing. I was so scared as I pulled my car off the road, and I called my sister in a panic. We knew there was something terribly wrong in my body since these symptoms kept lingering and wouldn't go away, so we agreed I would call the ambulance to get me. Surely with all the heart monitors and tests the hospital could run, I'd get answers.

Unfortunately, they still couldn't find any physiological reasons for the way I felt. The chest pains were an even bigger wake-up call to dig deeper and understand what was going wrong with my health. This question forced me to do thorough research on my own. I was eating healthy foods, sleeping well, taking time for myself, focused on my purpose, and managing my emotions not to impact my body, and still, something was wrong.

But the point here is that I tried EVERYTHING to get my health under control. And when I reached my rock bottom where my symptoms got so bad that I called an ambulance, it's like it was a gift from above. I feel like that hospital visit happened to put me on a path to find the last piece to the puzzle that I had been looking for.

There was another element of a healthy lifestyle that wasn't about what I did, but it was something happening to me. Finally, I found the missing piece when I decided to be my own doctor. I learned a lot about toxicity and pathogens from Anthony Williams, The Medical Medium. He teaches that toxins fuel viruses and make them stronger. So, I had to work on eliminating the toxins in my environment in order to take away the trigger that was making the virus grow stronger. Thus, the missing link had to be the environmental toxicity—and sure enough, I was right! I did exhaustive searches on the internet and learned that there's an entire set of research and information about how toxicity in our bodies and environments can also cause symptoms like mine.

Most likely, environmental toxicity is new news for you, as it was for me, too. Consider this. You already know that air pollution can impact your health, especially if you're already vulnerable and have asthma—and even if you don't, when that pollution is bad enough, it can make anyone ill. Air pollution is mostly invisible, and you might not even smell it, but it can be monitored and measured. Take what you already know then, and let's imagine for a second that those known pollutants in the air are just a small tip of the overall amount of toxins that can be present in your environment and have an impact on your body.

Finally, I consulted a naturopath because most medical doctors aren't taught about toxins unless they seek it out themselves. The naturopath helped me find out exactly what was wrong. For me, the mystery symptoms that were plaguing me for 3 1/2 years came down to two things:

1. Pathogens - these are bugs (& in my case, this was viral).

2. Toxins - so things like heavy metals, plastics, chemicals, pesticides, etc.

Let's start with Pathogens. I had a virus called HHV6. Essentially, that meant I had something in my body compromising my immune system and making me have chronic fatigue, and I had no idea it was there. I had been fighting a totally uphill battle against an unknown enemy and with no help from my doctor who also had no idea. Then, my body also had toxins I was storing that interfered with my nervous system and natural processes. To feel better, I had to find a way to heal myself so I could bring my body back into balance with my total wellness.

These two things were contributing to my symptoms and the missing link to *why* I wasn't feeling my best. No disrespect, but over the last few years I have really come to realize how flawed our healthcare system is. Many doctors will often treat the symptoms - by giving us a drug, which produces a side effect, which then contributes to toxicity in the body—and then further contributes to more ill health. That's certainly what my experience was.

I was always aware that toxins were harmful, like we think about air pollution, but I guess I never took it seriously until I experienced the effects firsthand - and boy can it be debilitating. The problem is that there are literally toxins everywhere we go, and we can't escape them. I remember booking a spontaneous holiday to Cancun with my family because I was desperately craving a vacation to escape the freezing temperatures in Toronto. I needed the healing benefits of the sun. But I couldn't believe the amount of toxins there was all around us during the trip. From the sprays the landscaper was using on the grass, to the heavy-duty perfume in the lobby and washrooms – I couldn't escape it.

This is not to say that we're doomed. There are many protective measures we can take, and that's what we do in our own home. I made it my mission to turn my home into my sanctuary (but I did this slowly, as doing everything 'all at once' can be overwhelming).

LESSON LEARNED

The biggest piece to this puzzle was learning that the majority of my symptoms ultimately had to do with environmental toxicity. It was the trigger to the various neurological symptoms I was experiencing.

I did a toxicity test that told me I had high levels of chlorine from the water I was drinking and other chemicals from my mattress and heavy metals. That can come from food, water, and the air, and it brings havoc to your brain and body systems. In order to heal, I used my infrared sauna to detox and drink fresh water to flush out the toxins, as well as removing many other toxins from my home.

Even if you don't have an infrared sauna, there are a lot of changes you can make in your home to decrease the toxins. Here are some tips from Amy Meyers, MD's "Healthy Cookware Guide" for your kitchen (available at www.AmyMeyersMD.com). There can be toxicity in the chemicals that make up your cleaning products, so start switching the ones with labels that have things you can't pronounce to something clean and more natural. Also, if you have ceramic-coated and Teflon pans, switch to ones with enamel cast iron or stainless steel. If this idea is overwhelming, start making one change a week until you've completely detoxed your kitchen, then do the same thing with the personal care and cleaning products in your bathroom.

There are also electro-pollution factors all around us, which come from electromagnetic fields due to high electricity voltages and Wi-Fi, and more. To limit your exposure and make your home electro-pollution free, Meyers has some easy suggestions: don't use the Bluetooth on your phone, use speaker phone instead of holding your cell to your head, turn off your Wi-Fi router at night, and avoid resting your devices against your body when using them.

There are also foods that help you detox. In addition to everything in my chapter on food, you can drink filtered water with freshly squeezed lemon in the mornings, cucumber juice in the evenings and eat more leafy greens. Check out Anthony Williams's books, as well as radio shows and his website, www.MedicalMedium. com, for many recipes and specific foods that will help you clear toxins from your body.

Sometimes the best thing you can do is make your body a natural detox machine because we can't avoid 100% exposure outside the home, even when your home is detoxed as much as you possibly can.

HEALTHY LIFESTYLE ALIGNMENT

Once I understood that I had an unknown pathogen and toxins built up in my body, I was able to make changes to my environment and my health to get back into balance. If you've ever felt like you "just want to feel like yourself again," and nothing else is working, but you know something is wrong, you might want to look at possible toxins that are sabotaging your healthy habits.

We can't address what we don't understand, so when you don't get good answers from doctors, don't give up on yourself, as I didn't. Once you know what's really wrong, you can adapt as needed to detox and get back in alignment with your wellbeing.

IDEAS FOR DETOXIFICATION

<u>Rebounder</u>

Oxygen has positive effects on our nervous system. A great way of getting more oxygen into my system was jumping on my rebounder for 5-10 minutes per day. By doing this exercise, every cell gets massaged so waste materials then gets squeezed out. Our lymph system is what carries waste and when we're bouncing around it gets the lymph moving which helps to eliminate toxins.

<u>Infrared Sauna</u>

Skin is our largest organ. The sauna is fantastic as it allows us to shed toxins. The effects of this on my mental state were massive – wow! My skin would glow, and the treatment gives me that surge of energy I needed when I feel low. I use this literally everyday, whether going first thing in the morning for a fresh start to my day, after a workout or just before bed to relax and call it a day.

<u>Hydration</u>

The more hydrated you are, the more you're detoxing! I start my day with 16 oz of filtered water and freshly squeezed lemon and then aim to have another glass in the afternoon. This is one of my favourite routines because my head feels clear, and the fogginess is gone.

<u>Dry Brushing</u>

Since the skin is the largest elimination organ – I decided to give this a go every single day (plus it's easy to do)! Because of the massaging effect of the bristles, it's highly effective at stimulating blood circulation and the lymphatic system, plus it eliminates toxins.

Massage

Massage stimulates the lymphatic system which helps to eliminate waste and toxins. I aimed for 1-2 massages/week. This can be expensive, so I looked at my overall expenses to see where I could cut back so I could put those funds towards massage instead.

Hot Yoga

You may have heard that you can "sweat out toxins" by doing a hot yoga class. After being overburdened by toxins, I was open to doing anything that helped me flush them out. Doing hot yoga forced me to drink more water because of how much I would sweat, which further accelerates the body's ability to detoxify more waste.

Epsom Salt Bath

Salt baths allow for minerals to draw out toxins from the body. This is something I would aim for in the evening as a "treat" before bed. This was a god sent as it killed two birds with one stone and helped with my insomnia too.

Reflection Questions

1. Are there any toxic things around your home that need to be tossed out and replaced? Make a list of things you want to work on.

2. Which detoxification protocols appeal to you most?

Happiness is the new rich.
Inner peace is the new success.
Health is the new wealth.
Kindness is the new cool.

- Syed Balhki

CHAPTER 8

• •

Final Thoughts

Until it happened to me and my health suffered, I didn't understand the saying, "prepare for impact because you never know what life will throw at you." These days, I don't take anything for granted, especially my health. I'm STILL in network marketing (money is still important, and I have a family). But getting to the next level and then the next level isn't my only focus anymore. I'm now growing and evolving as a person—that's my goal, instead of making 'more money' as my goal. it's not that wanting more financial freedom is wrong, but I learned that I can better align with wealth and success when I nurture myself from the inside out.

A big part of this has been getting my purpose out there, as Amber the psychic medium suggested. As soon as I started getting creative again (which is a value of mine) and started blogging, writing my book, putting my website up, etc., I started feeling like myself again. I had that spark, which has a direct impact on health and well-being. This change came after I neglected my creativity for years.

It was a big financial risk for me to step back from my network marketing business to take care of my health. Fortunately, I was in the only kind of business that I know of that you can build and then it can run on its own. So, during all this time I was looking for cures and making lifestyle changes, I still get monthly checks. How amazing is that?

I've done A LOT of reflecting and learning over the years, and what I can say from my experience is that network marketing is a brilliant business model. It's been so amazing that it allowed me to take three years off to:

- Rest heal & reclaim my health.
- Pay for alternative health care (because I refused to go to doctors whose only goal was to give me a drug to mask what's "really" going on).
- Go back to school for a year and follow my passion.
- Publish two books – writing became very therapeutic during this time!
- Go to multiple healers, practitioners, coaches, seminars to learn everything I could to be my own doctor.

When reflecting back on each chapter within this book - it's hard to believe I was doing the polar opposite of what I teach for so long. I wanted to be healthy and thought I was doing the right things, but I wasn't. Meanwhile, I truly 'thought' I was living a healthy lifestyle. I don't think I'm alone on this either. A lot of other people believe they are living a healthy lifestyle by following what they perceive to be 'healthy' - but they are not sleeping enough or practicing self care.

True vitality and wellbeing means looking at things holistically - not just looking at what you put on your plate, but off your plate too. Working on diet and lifestyle together is key. Remember the "primary foods" I discussed in the introduction? This is it. It's a nice balance of healthy food, sleep, self-care, purpose, emotions and detox.

And although it felt like my world was falling apart when my symptoms were at their worst, I learned that in order for things to get better, I needed to face fear right in the eye. That meant walking away from security and being okay with uncertainty. Because here's the thing – what we resist persists. So sometimes making those tough decisions and doing what's risky may be in our best interest. Because problems won't just disappear by pretending that they're not there.

There were too many things that I was doing everyday that didn't excite me anymore. And if I'm not happy then what's the point, right? Life is meant to be enjoyed. So, let me ask you. If time and money weren't an issue, what would you be doing with your life right now? And is it everything you are doing today? If not, what do you need to start doing that will bring you closer to your dreams?

Many of us are taught to just go through the motions. As if feeling tired, stressed and busy is a *normal* way of life. Or having a fancy title, position or degree is what makes someone *successful*. But success means different things to different people. I no longer felt successful if I didn't feel healthy and genuinely happy. This is what I want my kids to know right from the beginning and I wanted to pave that way for them so they could be proud and have a role model to follow.

Are you doing the work that you chose because you *want* to or because someone told you that you *should?* Oftentimes we feel that we should because it's a great paying job, it's secure and it's socially acceptable. But when we "should" on ourselves and it's not what we truly want deep down inside, we're not being honest about how we really feel because we're keeping our true feelings hidden. Most people don't realize how much more AMAZING life can be because we're so conditioned to think life should be 'okay!'

Walking away from something that's weighing us down takes courage. But if something doesn't feel right, the sooner we get rid of it, the sooner the right things will start to show up. Letting go always makes way for us to get closer to our truth. Otherwise, we give up precious space to something not precious to us. Getting as close to our authentic self as possible is where *living in the now* occurs. And fueling our body with love so we can get rid of any lingering negative emotions during this process!

So I made it my mission that as soon as I felt my BEST – I was going to spend the rest of my life learning all there is to know about holistic healthy living and helping others live a healthier lifestyle - from the *inside* out!

Moral of the story - prepare for impact. We just never know what life will throw at us. I truly believe that everyone should be working on an additional income stream (especially one that pays residuals) - whether that's in Network Marketing or something else. There's nothing more freeing than choosing NOT to trade your time for a paycheck - should something unexpected come your way.

I hope this book had a positive impact on your vitality & well-being. If it did, it would mean so much to me if you recommend it to others.

With love,

Deborah Xo

ABOUT THE AUTHOR

Deborah has been a network marketer for the last decade and has inspired hundreds of leaders to create a lifestyle of freedom through network marketing. She has achieved remarkable success and has been recognized for various top-level awards. She is also a certified Life & Health Coach and has appeared in publications, such as *Thrive Global* and *Fit after 45*.

Deborah is a wife and mother of two. When she's not spending time with her family, you can find her working out at the gym, reading a good book or travelling some place warm, of course. To learn more, please visit www.deborahlobart.com

RESOURCES

Meyer, Amy. www.AmyMyersMD.com

The Institute for Integrative Nutrition: www.IntegrativeNutrition.com

Williams, Anthony. www.MedicalMedium.com

Williams, Anthony. *Life-Changing Foods: Save Yourself and The Ones You Love with The Hidden Healing Powers of Fruits and Vegetables.* Carlsbad, Hay House, Inc. 2016.

Wilson, Sarah. of *I Quit Sugar: Your Complete 8-Week Detox Program and Cookbook* New York City, Clarkson Potter. 2014.